Ketogenic Diet for Beginners

The Most Effective Guide for Rapid Weight Loss

Table Of Contents

Chapter 1 – What is the ketogenic diet?

The ketogenic diet is a specific medical regime, which was primarily used in order to treat epileptic seizures in children. This diet is based on a high fat content, with low levels of protein and carbohydrates. Even though it was at first recommended in epileptic children, nowadays it is often recommended for those who are interested in losing weight. Given the low carb content of this diet, the body is practically forced to burn fat, which ultimately leads to the desires weight loss.

In a normal diet, the carbohydrates obtained from the ingested foods are transformed into glucose. The glucose is distributed then throughout the entire body, fueling different organs and guaranteeing their normal functioning (including the brain). The carbohydrates are broken down in the liver; however, if the body receives reduced quantities of carbohydrates, fat is going to be converted by the liver into fatty acids and ketone bodies. These ketone bodies are actually the basis of the ketogenic diet; as they reach vital organs, such as the brain, they become energy fuel instead of the glucose. The initial research made on the ketogenic diet what based on the idea that the increased levels of ketone bodies are responsible for the reduced epileptic seizures.

From that research, it was just a step to discover the benefits of the ketogenic diet for those who were trying to lose weight. The research had already shown that this diet provided the body with enough quantities of proteins and carbohydrates, promoting weight loss through the burning of fat. This was the start of one of the most popular diets out there, with the classical ketogenic diet respecting the 4:1 or 3:1 ratio (fat to protein and carbohydrates).

One of the main ideas behind the ketogenic diet is to exclude the foods that have high carb content, such as bread, pasta, grains or sugar. The diet is also based on the exclusion of fruits and vegetables with similar starch content. While lowering the consumption of foods that are rich in carbs or proteins, the ketogenic diet promotes the increased consumption of foods that are rich in fat, such as different types of nuts, cream or butter. As you will have the opportunity to discover in this book, there are several variants of the ketogenic diet. A particular example will be the MCT (medium-chain triglycerides) ketogenic diet, in which half of the calories are accounted for by using a special coconut oil (rich in MCT).

The ketogenic diet was invented by a doctor (Russell Wilder), at the Mayo Clinic, somewhere around 1924. In the past few years, it made a comeback, being often chosen for the weight loss benefits that are offered. However, there are a few things that you need to keep in mind when it comes to this particular diet. The first and most important thing is that medical supervision is a must; this diet is followed under the specialized advice and assistance of a trained technician. Second of all, it requires a lot of work and hours put into it, with food being measured and weighed for each and every meal.

The control of the caloric intake is required for the success of the ketogenic diet. It is also important to take vitamin and mineral supplements, so as to compensate for those absent from the diet. In the past, the intake of fluids was restricted in the ketogenic diet. Today, thanks to the current research, the fluids are no longer restricted in this particular diet. Studies performed on the patients who have followed such a diet have shown that the lack of fluids can impair the functioning of the kidneys, leading to kidney stones among other modifications.

The ketogenic diet is adapted to each person, following a clear and specific structure, with well-chosen meal plans. As it was already mentioned, the food for each meal is weighed and it is recommended that the person consumes all the food on the plate for the best results (the more fats are ingested, the more extensive the burning of those fats is going to be in the liver). It has also been used as a low glycemic therapy, helping patients who are suffering from diabetes and other similar health problems to keep their glucose levels under control.

The calories that are drawn from the carbohydrate intake in the standard diet are between 45% and 65% of the total amount. With the ketogenic diet, the carbohydrate intake is reduced, so as to represent only between 2% and 4% of the total amount. Also, it is important to remember that the ketogenic diet is a high fat diet, not a high protein diet. On the contrary, the protein intake is kept down to a constant low level, so as to maintain the health of the body.

The ketones or ketone bodies that result from the break down of the ingested food are actually replacing the glucose, being the alternative fuel that is going to promote weight loss. One must remember that these ketone bodies reduce the systemic inflammation that is commonly encountered in epilepsy and other neurodegenerative diseases; at the same time, they promote the weight loss process, in a health manner (not as it happens with other weight loss program, when a person practically starves in order to lose weight).

As a beginner into the world of the ketogenic diet, there are a lot of things that you need to learn about the way this diet works. In the following chapter, you will be presented with information on the health benefits of the ketogenic diet. You can then move on to the next chapter and read about the ketogenic diet food list, discovering the foods that you are allowed to eat and the ones you should avoid. The following chapter is dedicated to the four variants of the ketogenic diet, while the last chapter concentrates on how to lose weight using this amazing diet. Enjoy your journey into the wonderful universe of the ketogenic diet!

Chapter 2 – Health benefits of the ketogenic diet

The ketogenic diet can be a powerful tool that can change your life. Switching to a diet that is very low in carbohydrates, in which the fat gets converted to energy, can help to reduce high blood pressure, relieve your heartburn and pain in the joints, and to stop the pre-diabetic condition.

The ketogenic diet contains high proportions of fat, a moderate amount of protein and very little carbohydrates, and was used in medicine primarily to treat difficult kontolirajuće epilepsy in children. The diet mimics aspects of starvation by forcing the body to burn fat instead of carbohydrates. Into common circumstances, carbohydrates contained in food are converted into glucose, which is then transmitted through the body, and this is especially important in stimulating brain function. However, if there is very little carbohydrate in the diet, the liver will convert fat into fatty acids and ketone bodies. They enter the brain and replace glucose as an energy source. Elevated levels of ketones in the blood, a condition known as ketosis, lead to a reduction in the frequency of epileptic seizures.

This method has been used since 1920's and through the next decade when its popularity fell by the introduction of anticonvulsant drugs, which is a typical situation showing the pharmaceutical industry imposes instead of natural ways for solving problems.

When you start with this diet, your body goes through several adjustments. After about two days from the start of the diet, the body starts to use ketones. In this way, the body rapidly loses weight, primarily fat. Muscle mass remains relatively unchanged because the diet contains, as stated, moderate amounts of protein.

In this diet, the prevalent foods are rich in protein, such as cheese, eggs, meat and fish. All of these foods contain very few carbohydrates. In addition, it is very important to eat vegetables in sufficient amounts, due to the high amount of fibers, vitamins and other essential substances for the body. Some vegetables contain large amounts of carbohydrates and these foods should be avoided, for example potatoes, rice, beans, peas, etc. Instead, you should consume cucumbers, cabbage, lettuce and other similar vegetables.

According to the Ketogenic Diet Resource website, the ketogenic diet is not a high protein diet, contrary to popular belief.

Some medical researchers and doctors use the Ketogenic diet for:

- Getting the cancer cells into remission with a new and effective means of treating cancer
- Treating epilepsy with the outcome being a reduction or even complete elimination of the attacks
- Helping patients with Alzheimer's disease to improve memory and brain functions
- Better control of the blood sugar for the people with diabetes
- Elimination of gluten allergy symptoms and alleviating the symptoms of other allergic reactions associated with autoimmune reactions
- Ketogenic diet helps various kidney diseases

The weakness of the kidney is a major complication caused by diabetes, but a US study on mice showed that a low-carb diet and with a lot of fat can correct this disorder within two months. This diet is so restrictive that it should be implemented with the help of experts. The meal, for example, may consist of fried eggs with sour cream, omelet with bacon and buttered lettuce or abundantly watered mayonnaise. A person gets largely deprived of carbohydrates and sugar, when this diet is used. The body uses the fat instead glucose for burning energy. In this way, the diabetics will block the glucose toxic effects - simple sugars that the body produces during food metabolism. This sugar is harmful for diabetics because they do not have enough insulin to regulate it.

An American team at the New York Mount Sinai hospital has done research on two groups of mice that were genetically predisposed to have diabetes type 1 or type 2 diabetes. Half of the mice were fed standard, food rich in carbohydrates, while the other half was subjected to ketogenic diet. After eight weeks, kidney weakness is neutralized in mice that were fed according to the katogenic diet principles.

Charles Mobs, the team leader of the research once said that this study shows that diabetes can be stopped just by making changes to the diet. According to the US National Institutes of Health, there are over 24 million people with diabetes in the United States, of which nearly 180,000 suffer from renal failure, as a result of the disease. Mobs points out that ketogenic diet probably is not suitable as a long-term solution, but it seems that using it the whole life is not needed, because only one month of such food is enough to do a “body reset" in order to help the failure of the kidneys.

He also notes that his team's findings point to the possibility of developing new drugs and pharmacological agents that would eventually produce the same effects as a strict implementation of the ketogenic diet. The team from Mount Sinai is planning to conduct new studies to investigate the impact of the aforementioned diet on other neurological diseases, among other things, on retinopathy, which causes loss of vision.

The ketogenic diet delivers numerous other health benefits, as you will have the opportunity to discover below. By reading the following paragraphs, you will gain more knowledge about the advantages that the ketogenic diet brings in terms of health.

These are the claimed health benefits of the ketogenic diet:

- Reduction of appetite
    - You can follow the diet without feeling hungry all the time
    - Allows you to consume fewer calories
    - No effort to cut back, no temptation to give up
- Weight loss
    - The ketogenic diet will help you lose more weight in a shorter amount of time
    - Diuretic properties – removal of excess water in the body (the foods that you eat will lower the

insulin levels, allowing the kidneys to excrete the excess sodium and promoting the fast weight loss process)
    - Maximum efficiency – first six months
- No more belly fat
    - Reduction of abdominal fat – known for its negative consequences over one's health (especially cardiovascular risks)
    - Reduced risk of cardiovascular disease and type 2 diabetes
    - The metabolism is activated once again, burning abdominal fat
- Reduction of triglycerides
    - As this diet is low in carbs, you will experience a reduction in the triglycerides levels (normally associated with cardiovascular disease and other health problems)
- Increased level of HDL (good cholesterol)
    - Lower risk of cardiovascular disease
- Reduction of blood sugar levels
    - The low carb content of the ketogenic diet allows for the insulin levels to be kept under control, especially in patients who have already been diagnosed with type 2 diabetes

  - When followed under specialized assistance, the ketogenic diet can replace the medication that one normally takes in order to lower the insulin levels
- Constant blood pressure
  - The ketogenic diet can reduce the increased blood pressure, protecting the person against cardiovascular disease but also against other health problems, such as stroke or kidney failure
- Ketogenic diet – treatment for metabolic syndrome
  - Metabolic syndrome includes a number of symptoms, including the presence of excess abdominal fat, hypertension, hyperglycemia, increased triglycerides levels and reduced levels of good HDL cholesterol
  - The ketogenic diet can effectively be used as a treatment for the metabolic syndrome, reducing the associated risks of cardiovascular disease and diabetes
- Reduced size of LDL (low density lipoprotein) molecules – 'bad cholesterol'
  - The ketogenic diet is poor in carbohydrates, which leads to a change in the size of the LDL molecules

    - As the LDL molecules go from large to small, the risk of cardiovascular disease is considerably reduced
- Ketogenic diet – treatment for epilepsy and other disorders of the brain (Parkinson's disease, Alzheimer's disease)
    - The ketogenic diet does not deliver glucose to the brain, but ketone bodies (thus preventing and reducing the frequency of epileptic seizures)
    - Recent studies are performed in order to determine whether the ketogenic diet could be used in other disorders of the brain, especially the neurodegenerative ones such as Parkinson or Alzheimer
- Control over eating habits
    - By reducing the carb intake, the cravings for glucose-based foods are going to disappear, offering thus a better control over one's eating habits
    - You can say goodbye to different food fixations you had in the past
    - No more craving for something sweet
- Decreased levels of CRP (C Reactive Protein) and HbA1c proteins

    - The ketogenic diet will lead to a decrease in the levels of the above mentioned proteins in the blood
    - Health benefit – reduced risk of heart disease (these proteins are markers of heart disease risk and inflammation in different parts of the body)
- Increased energy levels
    - Disappearance of chronic fatigue symptoms
    - You will feel more energized, prepared to handle every day activities with a renewed force
- No more muscle stiffness or pain in the joints
    - The ketogenic diet excludes grains among other foods from the diet, these being believed to be responsible for stiff muscles or stiff joints
- Say goodbye to the 'foggy' brain
    - A diet that is rich in carbs provides too much glucose for the brain, causing it to become foggy and your cognitive functions to be impaired
    - The ketogenic diet will help you think clear once again, your brain working at its full capacity
- Better sleeping habits
    - The ketogenic diet has a positive effect whereas the sleeping habits are concerned
    - Improvement of symptoms related to sleep apnea

  - The reduced carb intake allows for symptoms such as heartburn and increased blood sugar to disappear
  - No more daytime sleepiness or naps during the day
- Improvement or disappearance of GERD symptoms (heartburn)
  - Ketogenic diet – no grains or sugar – no GERD symptoms (especially heartburn, which can wake you from your sleep every night)
- Better oral health
  - A diet that is rich in sugar often leads to oral health problems, such as cavities, tooth decay or gum disease
  - The ketogenic diet contributes to an improvement of the oral pH, thus protecting against oral health problems
- Improved digestion
  - The ketogenic diet helps one person have healthy digestion, having a positive effect whereas the bowel movements are concerned
  - Say goodbye to feeling bloated or gassy
  - No more abdominal pain or cramps
  - All due to the elimination of sugar and grains from the diet

- No more mood swings
    - The ketogenic diet delivers increased quantities of ketone bodies (broken down from the food) and these are effective in keeping important neurotransmitters such as serotonin and dopamine stable
    - Better mood control – one of the big health benefits of the ketogenic diet
- Protection against cancer
    - The ketogenic diet is low in sugar – sugar is believed to be one of the risk factors associated with the appearance of cancerous growths
    - By switching to the ketogenic diet, one can lower the risk of different types of cancer.

Chapter 3 – Ketogenic diet food list

With any diet, there are certain foods that are allowed to eat and others that you are forbidden from touching. Knowing which foods are allowed and which foods you should avoid in the ketogenic diet will make your life easier, so do not hesitate to check out the ketogenic diet food list.

These are the foods you are allowed to include in your ketogenic diet:

- Fats and oils
    - Fish – good source of Omega3 and Omega6
    - Fish supplements – recommended to those who are not so crazy about fish
    - Saturated and monosaturated fats
        - Butter
        - Macadamia nuts
        - Avocado
        - Egg (yolk part)
    - Vegetable oils – only those that are cold-pressed
        - Olive
        - Soybean
        - Flax
        - Safflower

        - Red palm
    - For fried food
        - Non-hydrogenated lards
        - Beef tallow
        - Ghee
        - Coconut oil
    - Other recommended foods in this category include:
        - Chicken fat
        - Mayonnaise – recommended choice: homemade (the store bought kind often contains carbs, which should represent a low percentage of the ketogenic diet)
        - Coconut and peanut butter (especially the one that is made from macadamia nuts)
- Proteins
    - Fish – several choices were already presented above but you can also consider halibut, mackerel or cod
    - Seafood – great source of proteins – recommended choices: oysters, lobsters, crabs, mussels
    - Eggs – try to buy them from a farm (organic)
    - Meat – the most recommended source of protein – you can choose any kind of meat (with

red meat, try to choose beef that has been gras fed – healthier, increased quantities of fatty acids)

- Vegetables (preferably organic)
  - The list of allowed vegetables is long, including: asparagus, avocado, broccoli, carrots, cauliflower, celery, cucumber, garlic, green beans, mushrooms, onion (green and white), bell pepper, pickles, lettuce (romain, butterhead), shallots, peas, spinach, squash, tomato
- Dairy products (only a few are allowed in the ketogenic diet, as you will have the opportunity to discover below – always choose the ones that are made from organic milk)
  - Heavy whipping cream, sour cream and cottage cheese
  - Hard and soft cheeses
    - Cheddar
    - Mozzarella
    - Cream cheese
    - Mascarpone
- Nuts and seeds
  - Recommended in reduced quantities
  - Selected choices

        - Macadamia
        - Walnuts
        - Almonds
    - Other recommended choices include:
        - Chia seeds
        - Flax seeds
        - Pumpkin seeds
        - Sesame seeds
        - Sunflower seeds
    - Can also be used as flour, instead of the regular kind (for baking purposes)
- Beverages
    - Water – most recommended (no limit to how much one is allowed to drink)
    - Unsweetened tea – preferably herbal (not black, no sugar)
    - Artificial sweeteners might be allowed, in order to help you control your cravings for sugar (liquid sweeteners are recommended in moderate quantities, as these do not contain carbs)
- Spices
    - Moderate consumption is recommended – they contain sugar and carbs, which are not indicated in the ketogenic diet

  - Allowed: sea salt, pepper (black, cayenne), oregano, basil, chili (powder), parsley, cilantro, turmeric, thyme, sage, rosemary

These are the foods that you should avoid or reduce in regard to your ketogenic diet:

- Hydrogenated fats
  - Margarine – increased risk of heart disease
  - Not the kind of fats that are recommended to be included in the ketogenic diet
- Increased quantities of:
  - Almonds
  - Walnuts
  - Pine nuts
  - Cashews
  - Pistachio
  - Different types of oil – sunflower oil, corn oil (high content of Omega 6 – increased risk of inflammation in different parts of the body)
- Certain spices (because of the carbohydrates content)
  - Onion or garlic powder
  - Bay leaves
  - Cinnamon
  - Ginger
  - Allspice

    - Cardamom
- Fruits (because of the increased sugar levels)
    - Fruits that should be especially avoided – raspberries, cranberries, blueberries
- Store-bought tomato sauce (increased sugar levels)
- Diet soda – even though it contains artificial sweeteners, it will increase your appetite for sugar.

Cheeses are not exactly the ideal food for the keto diet as full-fat cheeses often have a lot of hidden carbs, so they should be consumed only in very small quantities. Many supporters of the keto diet are against cream and cottage cheese as well, despite the fact that these types of cheese are low in carbs. Still, every cheese and, in fact, every dairy product contains lactose and you need to get your carbs only from fiber, not any type of sugar.

You have been presented with the foods that you are allowed to eat and those that should be avoided while you are following the ketogenic diet. However, this food list will not help you control your cravings – for this, you will need to read the below paragraphs. By reading, you will have the opportunity to discover how to keep your craving under control, replacing your cravings with healthy choices.

Chocolate is one of the most often encountered cravings but, in reality, what your body asks for is magnesium. So, instead of eating chocolate, you can satisfy the need for magnesium by eating different nuts or seeds (in moderate quantities). Another big craving is represented by sweets – in this case, your body might be asking for different things, including chromium, carbon or phosphorus. For chromium, eat broccoli or cheese; for carbon, the best choice is spinach, whereas for phosphorus, you can either eat chicken, beef or eggs. If you have a craving for bread or pasta, this means your body actually needs nitrogen – satisfy your craving by consuming a nice piece of red meat. The craving for salty foods is based on the body requiring chloride or silicon, which can be obtained by consuming fish or nuts/seeds.

Glucose and all of the carbohydrates in general, are not used in fat-rich diets, because they bring the body out of ketosis. The most important thing about ketogenic diet is being careful not to ingesting glucose through some sort of cheese or vegetables that contain way too many carbohydrates. The essence of this diet is accepting a totally different diet approach than the one you're used to. When the ketonic diet brings the results, people find it hard to stop with the diet.

It is important to note that this diet doesn't require too much money. In fact, there aren't many diets that can save you money like the ketonic diet. It would be smart of you to invest the saved money into buying sport supplements. Whey powder contains a fair amount of carbohydrates but if you take it during the workout, you will burn them easily. Probably the best way to improve the amount and quality of the protein in your diet is to buy a BCAA powder or glutamine powder. Both of these supplements will help you retain the muscle mass, while burning the fat.

After the first two weeks, you can start the so-called creatine charging. Take at least 30 garms of creatine powder throughout the day and about 10 grams of glutamine. Glutamine would be smart taking after each workout, and before bed. The fat diets won't make you lose strength, but taking some fat burner more as a stimulant before the training is recommendable. It is known that thermogenics work better on fatty diets, so using a fat burner as well, can make wonders.

Caffeine is also a good way of increasing energy levels. Doses of about 200 mg before the training will help you feel invigorated and in the mood to hit the gym hard. Actually, caffeine will also help you burn fat as this substance improves the metabolism. However, you must be careful as large doses of caffeine can have negative effects on the body.

Some authors like King Body Opus even experimented with insulin in order to get into ketosis as soon as possible, which is really crazy and not recommended. But, let's say that people who care for health will take alpha lipolic acid in order to improve insulin sensitivity and get a better muscle pump, without putting on excessive fat.

In any ketogenic / anabolic / Atkins / fatty diet, it is not essential that you are in ketosis (nor you need keto sticks to show that you are in ketosis). its highest advantage is that the insulin is constantly low. As insulin is the one hormone that blocks the lipolysis (the use of body fat for energy), keeping it low is very important. Another advantage is that the excess ketones cannot be stored in the body, but are ejected through urine, sweat, etc. When you work or even when you're sitting, thinking, the body uses fat to produce energy.

The body "switches" glucose with ketones in producing energy, when a high fat intake is going on. That means that is about 50 to70% of total calories comes from fat and the carbohydrate intake is extremely low (around 30-50 grams per day), the body will start burning the body fat. The amount depends on the amount of muscle exercisers, so a body with a high percentage of muscle and "fast" metabolism can go with daily intake of 100 g of carbs. Keto sticks do not need to be used, because they are not accurate. For example, if you take a break for a while and measure the ketones, the sticks will show that you came out of ketosis. If the intake of carbohydrates is about 30 grams per day, the diet will work. The advantage of high fat intake is that you will never feel hungry like on a classic diet. Still, it's not the same when you stuff yourself with pastries, but fatty foods will make you feel full.

An additional advantage of the ketogenic diet is that it is more anabolic than conventional diets and practically, you can "get away" with less anticatabolics than in the classic diet, meaning that there is no chance you will lose muscle weight, only fat. Taking enough amounts of fat will slow down the release of amino acids from proteins in the bloodstream, so your body will have a high dose of amino acids all the time during the day, which is of course always the most important thing, not only for fitness but also for a proper brain function. The truth is, it always better to throw in an extra BCAA, glutamine and whey powder. It can hurt, but will make your muscle volume intact. But again, it is not necessary to take in abnormal quantities of protein and BCAA powder - approximately 30 grams not throw you out of ketosis.

A small disadvantage of the keto diet was found by bodybuilders. Muscle pump during this period is reduced. It can be solved by inserting creatine in the diet, or even better, adding a certain NO booster with no carbs. This supplement is best used right before training.

During the keto diet it is essential to add salted foods for the simple reason that due to restricted carbs amount, nothing will hold the water in the body. Practically, when you're on such a diet, if you don't take enough sodium, you will to the toilet every five minutes and water in the body during exercise is particularly important for the normal functioning of the joints, especially during the weight training.

If you already have quite a lot of muscle mass, but want to get rid of the fat on the stomach and other parts, you probably want to get on a cutting cycle. If you decide to use the keto diet for this, you probably want to make sure your muscles stay intact. They will, but the people assume they are getting smaller and thinner with every pound lost. So to avoid the negative effect on your view of your body, you might want to consider using some sport supplements. The old-school creatine should be your number 1 choice. This supplement has virtually no side effects and has plenty of benefits for your body, but not just for the muscle, for your brain and heart as well. Creatine also helps your hair grow and some studies have shown it does well to your skin. One thing is certain, creatine will give your muscles a bulk, a better blood flow, which will then lead to increased strength. So, hit hard on the gym and say hello to creatine.

The basic variant of creatine is monohydrate, which has been in use for decades by professional bodybuilders like Arnold Schwarzenegger, on a daily basis. However, in the recent couple of years, supplement companies have developed advanced versions of creatine. There are some NO reactors that contain several types of creatine mixed together in a perfect way, which will produce amazing results. These powders also contain vitamins and minerals, while some of them have a high content of caffeine as well. So, be sure not to take too much of it before bed.

Chapter 4 – Ketogenic diet variants

The ketogenic diet is available in different variants, each with its own set of rules and advantages to offer. These four variants are: classic ketogenic diet, MCT oil ketogenic diet, modified Atkins and low glycemic index treatment. Below, you will find a succinct presentation of each of these diet variants.

The **classic ketogenic diet** requires a structured meal plan to be realized by a trained and experience dietitian, taking into account the age, weight and activity levels of the person going on the diet. In establishing the meal plan for the ketogenic diet, one might also have to consider the cultural background and alimentary preferences. As it was mentioned in another chapter, the ratio of the ketogenic diet is 4:1 or 3:1 (fat to combined carb and protein levels). The protein levels are adjusted, so as to cover the necessities of each individual, whereas the carbohydrate levels are set according to the remaining allowance. The important thing is that the established ratio is maintained – this is the reason why the carbohydrate content in different medication or supplements is taken into consideration as well.

After the daily intake of fat, protein and carbohydrates has been established, the dietitian will proceed to dividing this intake among the main meals of the day. It is important that the person eats the entire meal, the snacks being included within the meal. There is also the ketocalculator, which can be efficiently used for generating various recipes. The basic principle of the classic ketogenic diet is that each meal includes these four components: cream (heavy whipping), meat (rich source of proteins), fruit/vegetable (only few selected fruits are allowed, as the majority have high sugar levels) and butter (source of fat). The food quantities for each meal are measured precisely, with the help of the electronic scale. Keep in mind that the classic ketogenic diet is not balanced; in order to remain healthy, a person will also have to take vitamin and mineral supplements.

The **MCT oil diet** is another variant of the ketogenic diet, being based on the usage of medium-chain triglycerides instead of low-chain triglycerides. Studies have shown that the MCT oil diet delivers more ketogenic effects than the one that is based on regular dietary fats (LCT). In this variant of ketogenic diet, 45% of the calories are derived from the MCT oil – this is lower than it was in the past but it offers a reduced risk for gastrointestinal complaints and ketogenic effects at the same time. A big advantage of the MCT oil diet is that it allows for the fat content to be reduced, while the protein and carb content can be increased. This automatically can be translated into the person following this diet having a wide array of food choices and being able to consume portions that are larger in size.

A third variant of the ketogenic diet is represented by the **modified Atkins diet.** If a person decides to follow this diet, there will be no limit on the calories or the proteins that are included in the daily meals. Apart from that, the followed ratio is of 1:1 and the diets do not necessarily have to be supervised by a trained dietitian. Nevertheless, it is still not a balanced diet, requiring the constant administration of vitamin and mineral supplements, as it happens in the classic ketogenic diet.

The fourth variant of the ketogenic diet is the **low glycemic index treatment**. This is often the preferred choice for those who need to keep their blood sugar levels under control. The main advantage of this ketogenic diet variant is related to the fewer restrictions imposed to the person following this diet – from the start, the person is allowed to consume a higher amount of carbohydrates than in the classic variant of the ketogenic diet. In following this diet, one does not have to use the electronic scale in order to weigh the food, nor rely on the professional assistance offered by an experienced dietitian.

Before you decide on a particular type of ketogenic diet, it is for the best that you visit a professional dietitian and assess your options together. Even if the dietitian will not provide further support for the diet, the advice offered at the start might prove out to be more than valuable.

Chapter 5 – How to lose weight by achieving optimal ketosis

One of the big benefits that the ketogenic diet brings is the one of weight loss. If you want to lose weight using the ketogenic diet, you also have to understand what optimal ketosis means. First of all, ketosis is the state in which the body functions almost entirely by burning high amounts of fat (hence, the weight loss).

Ketosis is a condition characterized by elevated concentrations of ketone bodies in the blood, which occurs when the liver due to energy needs converts fat into fatty acids and ketone bodies. Ketones are the by-products formed during the beta oxidation of fatty acids, where the fatty acid forms acetyl CoA (acetyl coenzyme A) entering the Krebs cycle. To ketosis usually occurs when the use of fatty acids for energy production is increased, for example when a body is lacking glucose during fasting.

The ketogenic diet replaces glucose with fat as the main fuel for the body, including when it comes to the brain (new fuel – ketone bodies). The ketone bodies are broken down from the ingested food in the liver, their production being stimulated by the low blood sugar levels. Research has demonstrated that, the lower the blood sugar levels are, the bigger the increase in the production of ketone bodies is going to be.

The state of optimal ketosis is reached when there are enough ketone bodies identified in the blood and the insulin levels are low – this is the state in which the highest amount of fat is burned, leading thus to an active weight loss process. The levels of ketone bodies in the blood can be measured with similar devices to the ones that are used for the measuring of glycaemia; a small needle will prickle your finger and, based on the sample of blood, you will be able to find out your blood ketone level. The most recommended time to measure the amount of ketone bodies in the blood is in the morning, on an empty stomach.

If you are interested in losing weight through optimal ketosis, there are a few things that you need to take into consideration. First of all, you have to avoid the most common source of carbohydrates, such as pasta, bread, rice, potatoes or different types of sweets; at the same time, you need to pay an equal amount of attention to the intake of proteins. The higher the amount of proteins consumed, the higher your glucose levels are going to be. Increased glucose levels lead to a spike in the insulin, which will ultimately have a negative effect on the state of optimal ketosis. The trick for losing weight is to consume higher quantities of fat (see the ketogenic food list once more), while eating reduced quantities of proteins and carbohydrates. When analyzing your eating habits, you also have to pay attention to the carbs that come from other sources, such as those that are contained in varied drugs or supplements you might be taking.

If this is the first time you are thinking about starting the ketogenic diet for weight loss purposes, it might be a good idea to get rid of all the temptations you have in your kitchen, particularly the one that are high in carbs. Once you have removed all the temptations, go out and do some shopping, using the ketogenic food list. As you have probably understood by now, the ketogenic diet does not require any special foods but you have to be attentive to the things you are buying. Restock the kitchen with the items present on the ketogenic food list and start learning how to cook. The ketogenic diet requires home cooked meals and you will need to increase the amount of time that you spend in the kitchen. If you have always wanted to learn how to cook, there is no better time than the present to engage in such activities.

The biggest temptation when starting a new diet is to constantly measure your weight, in order to see how much you have lost in a certain period of time. Even if weight loss is the reason why you have started the ketogenic diet, don't start measuring your weight immediately, obsessing on how much weight you have lost on a daily basis. Trying to measure each and every ounce of fat you have lost will literally drive you crazy; plus, there are fluctuations caused by the elimination of water, so you will not be able to tell accurately, from the start, how much you have lost.

Experts in the ketogenic diet recommend weekly measurements, as these reflect an accurate weight loss process. They also recommend that the measurements should be jotted down, so as one is able to follow the progress he or she has made. Instead of focusing on the actual weight that is being lost, they indicate that one should concentrate on the long-term health benefits that the ketogenic diet provides. In fact, whenever you are tempted to quit and abandon your ketogenic diet plan, think about health and you will have a powerful reason to stick with your diet.

It is just as important to remain consistent and not cheat, as straying from the ketogenic diet plan will cost you in time. A single cheat day will throw your entire plan in chaos and you will have to restart your diet, taking a long time to recover from the consequences. It is for the best that you follow the diet accordingly, incorporating any snacks into the actual meal plan. If you refrain from the in-between meals and snacks, your insulin levels will be reduced and your body will start using even more fat for fuel, contributing thus to the weight loss process.

After a while of keeping this diet, you will notice that you are sweating a lot. The subcutaneous water always disappears when you eat a large meal of carbs. The reason for this is that the body adapts to the new conditions and because there is no glycogen in the muscles, the body begins to retain water. This condition is, however, short-lived, a few days without cardio workout and a big meal with carbs, changes everything for the better.

When it comes to "charging" with carbs, this is primarily psychological in nature and is done to get you through the diet because, although the keto diet does not make you hungry, it is not the same sense of satiety when you eat a carb-opulent meal with consuming only fat and protein. Among other things, this is because carbs act on the secretion of serotonin (the so-called hormone of happiness) and many other hormones. That is why it is recommended to insert carbs during only one day each week. At the same time, you will get your body accustumed to this nutrient and will not disturb the metabolism of carbohydrates in the body, once you are over with the diet.

During the charge day, it is not crucial "recharge" glycogen reserve, because the body is working effectively with empty glycogen stores as well, without any problems. A good example for that are Eskimos, who throughout their whole life do not eat carbs, but just meat and fat, and their body and mind have been functioning normally. These people have practically no known heart diseases. So, when the "recharge" is on the schedule, the aim is always, to reduce the "damage" that a high intake of carbs makes, so it is better to insert only one meal rich with carbs that will keep you full for at least a couple of hours, then to stretch the carb recharge for a couple of days.

You should aim to keep the carb recharge as short as possible and consume carbs quicker, allowing the body to quickly switch to ketones. It is crucial to start the recharge with clean carbs (like rice, for example) and then, when your stomach is already full, switch to junk food, which of course, you cannot eat a lot, because your stomach is already full. A smart way for doing the recharge is to eat in the evening, just before the night's sleep. When you make your last meal of the day a carbohydrate-rich one, you will get an insulin kick, which will make you sleepy. However, if you do it during the day, you will just make your body craving for more carbohydrates.

The biggest problem is if you consume over 30-50 grams of carbs during the day on a keto diet, because otherwise the body will stop using ketones for energy. When your body switched to ketones, it works extraordinarily and you do not even need that much sleep. If you increase the amount of carbs, you will constantly feel unwell. If you feel tired, uninspired, or your libido is low, during the keto diet, you might be ingesting some hidden carbs that you are not aware of.

The aim of the keto diet is that during the removal of subcutaneous fat you lose as small amounts of muscle mass as possible. Also, this diet should simply make you not so hungry as compared to other diets, making it easy to endure. It does not matter cutting the number of calories as the keto diet primarily focuses on switching the fuel that your body uses, from glucoses to ketones. Those ketones that are not used as fuel will get out of the body through urine and sweat.

Of course, it is better to take foods rich in essential fatty acids as the source of fat, primarily nuts, because for the regeneration of muscle cells, both EFA and EAA are required, while saturated fats will not be used for that. The keto diet works also if the source of fat is saturated fatty acids, fat is fat, but it is much healthier to enrich the diet with unsaturated fatty acids than saturated, but under the condition that you avoid consuming carbs. If your major source of fat is saturated fatty acids, again, you don't have to worry about cholesterol. There will be no increase in cholesterol levels as this can happen only in the presence of carbs.

Chapter 5 – Why you are not losing weight on the ketogenic diet

If you are on the ketogenic diet but you are not losing weight, there may be a few reasons behind such problems. In case your tests results have shown that you haven't reached optimal ketosis, the problem might lie in the carb intake (too high). The first thing that you want to do is calculate your overall carb intake and, if you notice it to be too high, to decrease the daily intake. It is also recommended that you include coconut oil in your diet, as this contains health medium-chain triglycerides. Your body can digest these MCT, burning the fat that results from them and provide you with unbelievable energy levels. What actually happens is that the medium-chain triglycerides are converted in the liver – from the process result the ketone bodies that help you reach the desired state of optimal ketosis.

There is always the risk of not being aware of all the carbs you are eating – this happens when you are choosing a product based on the fact that it is sugar free, but you do not check the label to check out the carb content as well. Also, if you are cheating on your diet and snacking on forbidden foods, you should definitely find the explanation for why you are not losing weight.

The high protein intake can also be responsible for you not being able to lose weight and not reaching optimal ketosis. In case you are eating foods that have too much protein, your body will take all that excess protein and convert it into glycogen, affecting the optimal ketosis process. You also need to pay attention to the protein supplements you are taking, as these definitely add to the overall protein intake.

Artificial sweeteners and hidden sugar sources can be held responsible for your inability to lose weight on the ketogenic diet. Artificial sweeteners, such as aspartame and the sugar contained in alcohol can disrupt the optimal ketosis process, thus preventing you from losing weight. You should be very careful about the potential sources of artificial sweeteners or sugar – these are commonly found in gum or mints, not to mention a wide range of drugs, including the ever popular cough syrup.

If your test results have shown that you are in ketosis but you are still not losing weight, the reason might be a high intake of fat and thus of calories. The most important thing that you have to remember is that not all calories have the same quality – you cannot expect to put an equal sign between the calories coming from healthy foods and those that are obtained by eating foods that are rich in carbs or extensively processed. It is for the best what you keep a clear track of how much calories you consume on a daily basis and remember that fat brings two times the calories carbs and proteins bring. Experts in the ketogenic diet recommend that between 60 and 75% of your calories should come from fat and no more.

Avoid excess eating and remember that losing weight becomes increasingly difficult as you come closer to your goals. Try to eliminate stress and sleep as much as you can, as these can also impair your ability to lose weight.

For competitors in bodybuilding, fitness and similar sports, who are using the keto diet regime, the calorie ratio between fat and protein should be about 50:50. That means that if you weight 90kg, as you need 2-3 grams of protein per each kg of body mass, you will need to take in 180-270 grams of protein per day. Because fats have a higher caloric value than protein, to make it 50-50 ration, you need to eat between 80 and 120 grams of fat, daily. The amount of carbohydrates should stay as low as 30 grams per day.

Most people are familiar with the fact that for fat burning, some long-term moderate-intensity (60-70% of MHR) exercises are necessary. Surely, that prolonged exercising causes an intense physical fatigue, but a bigger problem for the majority of exercisers is the psychological fatigue. People get their morale shot down when they realize that it takes up to 60 minutes to spend in one of the aerobic activities (running, cycling, etc). A good alternative, even more favorable for fat burning is the HIIT training. HIIT training is essentially an interval training, which means that it is a series of short-term, intense cardio series with active break. Physical activity that is chosen depends on the ability of the trainees themselves, so the beginners can just walk. Such training is considered to be aerobic, but has elements of anaerobic training. Its duration can be from 5-30 minutes. Interval training is therefore an excellent choice for people who have limited time for physical activity. However, for the HIIT, a body needs carbs, so this does not go well with the keto diet. LI cardio is a much better option than HIIT.

If a person at such a diet wants to "accelerate" the burning of the body fat, an ideal variant would be to insert some sorts of low-intensity cardio. HIIT is not a good option, because for this type, the body needs carbs. LI cardio is an ideal way for losing fat during the keto diet. LI cardio is a way of training that focuses on low intensity activates. It includes predominantly simple activities whose action is constantly repeated (cyclic Extracurricular activities) and where the energy consumption during the workout remains at the same level.

These activities mainly involve things like fast walking, but it could be done also with and easy cycling, stepper, orbitreck, swimming, etc. Actaully all of the activities that we can operate continuously at about 60-65% of max heart rate can be a part of LI training. We know that fat is burned almost exclusively in aerobic conditions, i.e. in the presence of oxygen, therefore LI cardio obviously is perfectly suited as the best type of activity for fat burning.

This is probably the reason why everyone immediately catches for LI cardio blindly, not knowing that by training high intensity anaerobic conditions the body also loses fat, but unlike LI cardio, HIIT is not during spending so much fat during the training, but the main consumption of fat begins during the recovery period, after the workout. The "put-down" of fat then can last quite a long, from a few hours to even a whole day.

After stopping the LI cardio an "afterburn" of the calories doesn't happen. Instead, the body relatively quickly returns to homeostasis, since the low intensity training is not nearly as demanding on the body as HIIT and did not cause the same physiological changes in the body as that type of training. Well, someone will think, what about the famous early morning LI cardio on an empty stomach, because, apparently it's the best thing possible.

One of the most publicized things about LI workout is doing it in the morning on an empty stomach, which in theory, because of empty depot of glycogen, will increase the consumption of energy from fat during the workout. Tips for doing cardio in the morning on an empty stomach you have probably heard least hundreds of times if you have ever talked about losing body fat with a fitness enthusiast.

Studies have, however shown that this was not the case as many people insists, among whom some prominent fitness instructors and bodybuilders. Increased insulin levels due to the meal before training, is the thing that actually reduces the release of fatty acids by 22%, but oxidation of that fat, (conversion of fat to energy) remains virtually the same, regardless of the empty stomach or if you've eaten before or even during the activity. The differences were only noticed after 80-90 minutes of workout. However, not many people are ready to spend that much time in the morning, working out. Another bad thing about workouts on an empty stomach is the fact that it has a bad influence on the muscle muss. The body will search for energy not only in fat, but also in muscle tissue, thus starting the catabolism. Glutamine, BCAA or a simple whey powder could be helpful, but then again, the body faces another problem – you will use those supplements for energy and won't lose fat. That means that cardio workout on an empty stomach is not a good idea. Actually, this is useless, contrary what proponents of so-called wonder diets say, like the ones that recommend the OMG 6-week diet.

The point is that the level of training and aerobic activity reduces the negative impact on the reduced release of fat after a meal. During aerobic activities of higher intensity, no advantages were even after 90 minutes, irrespective of the reduced release of fats and the lower concentration of free fatty acids in the plasma. It seems that the cause of this is that then the body releases more free fatty acid than it can use them. Meaning that those excessive fats get back, during the process, into the fat tissue and thus, this advantage gets lost.

It was also shown that with aerobic activity, a relatively high percentage of burned free fatty acids comes from intramuscular fat, but not from the subcutaneous fat tissue, which is the one we all want to get rid of as it is the only fat tissue noticeable. Considering that the intramuscular fat has no effect on the appearance or health of the body, we come to the conclusion that the slow cardio is not the best solution as it is often said. To make matters worse, the longer we do such workout and aerobic endurance training and get in the shape, we increase the supplies of intramuscular fat and a larger and larger percentage of fat consumed, comes precisely from these intramuscular fat. It is proven that a higher thermo effect of training and increased oxygen consumption in recovery after a workout happens with a meal before as opposed to training on an empty stomach.

All this mentioned above really does not look as something why this low intensity cardio should be done early in the morning on an empty stomach, which had been so loudly emphasized. The Li training is nothing more effective if you do it at any other time of the day or after a meal. It is essential to be substantially consistent and do it on regular basis. In the extreme case, sacrificing yourself by not eating and getting up early to hit the cardio, is not worth it. A better result, you'll get by eating normally and training when it suits you the best.

So, to conclude, here are the advantages of low intensity training. But, remember, this will not do anything good for your body shape, nor for your health (both mental and physical), if you don't implement the keto diet as well.

Low intensity cardio is fairly easy to endure. Everyone can walk, run, swim, cycle or perform similar activity, without many problems. Actually, this type of fitness is good for everyone, including those with high blood pressure or similar diseases. The LI cardio training is almost irreplaceable for those obese people who due to health issues need to lose weight. This will not put a lot of pressure on your heart, which is why it is relatively safe, even for those with cardiac issues. Unlike HIIT and weight training, the low intensity training will not lead to fatigue. The body will easily get back in the shape, which is why this type of training can be done on a regular basis.

However, nothing is perfect, including the LI cardio workout. It really does take a lot of time. For best results, you will have to invest at least an hour every day. But, where is a problem, there is always a solution. A good idea is to use the LI cardio as a way of commuting. Instead of going to the work by bus or car, why not walk or go by bicycle. Another bad thing about the low intensity training is that it somewhat boring – you need to repeat the same movements for quite a long period. A solution for that is to listen to music or watch television if you have a room bike. Also, you can listen to podcast or audio books as the brain activity is increased during the workout, which can help you learn better.

48405887R00032

Made in the USA
San Bernardino, CA
24 April 2017